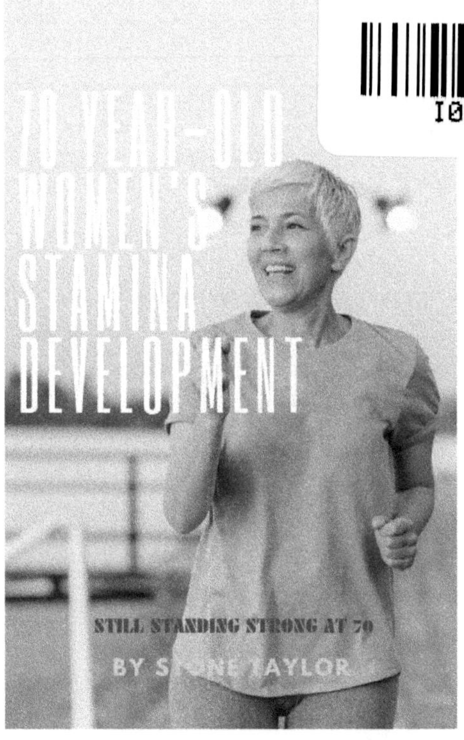

I0697286

STONE TAYLOR

TABLE OF CONTENT

· **CONCLUSION**

INTRODUCTION

It is natural for our physical qualities, notably our stamina, to deteriorate as we become older. For women in their 70s in particular, it is never too late to start working on enhancing our physical condition. In reality, regular exercise can help older women preserve their independence, lower their chance of developing chronic illnesses, and generally enhance their quality of life.

A thorough manual to assist women in their seventies build and maintain their stamina is available in the book "70-Year-Old Women's Stamina Development." This book offers helpful advice and exercises to assist older women reach their fitness objectives while addressing the individual physical and emotional problems they confront.

Understanding the aging process and how it affects stamina, fundamental exercise recommendations, the importance of nutrition, increasing cardiovascular endurance, strength training, yoga and Pilates, high-intensity interval training, mental stamina, and other issues are all covered in this book.

Women over the age of 70 can learn more about how to enhance their physical fitness and general health by reading this book. They may get the knowledge necessary to design a customised stamina development strategy and gain the confidence they need to take charge of their fitness and health. "70-Year-Old Women's Stamina Development" will help you achieve your objectives and enjoy the best possible health throughout your golden years, regardless of where you are in your fitness path or what new challenges you are searching for.

DEDICATION

I dedicate this book to old ladies who are at their 70 who desire to build their stamina stronger and stronger in order to have strong bones.

CHAPTER ONE

Maintaining the same degree of endurance and physical fitness that we did when we were younger might be difficult as we become older. The fact that our bodies may adapt and advance at any age must be understood, though. In this chapter, we'll talk about how to maintain your stamina as you get older and how to become in the best possible physical shape.

Knowledge of the Aging Process

Understanding how aging impacts our physical capabilities is crucial before we can talk about ways to increase stamina as we age. Our bodies change as we age in a number of ways that may affect our endurance, including:

Loss of muscle mass: As we become older, we lose muscle, which can make it more difficult to exercise and can lower our stamina.

Reduced cardiovascular function: As we age, our circulatory system's capacity to provide oxygen to our muscles reduces, which may have an impact on our endurance.

Decreased lung capacity: As we become older, our lung capacity declines, which can make it more difficult to breathe while exercising and reduce our stamina.

Less flexibility: As we age, our joints stiffen, making movement more difficult and lowering our stamina.

Increasing Your Endurance

There are several techniques to increase your stamina as you age despite these changes. These are some crucial tactics to take into account:

Establish a baseline: It's critical to gauge your current level of stamina before beginning any fitness regimen. You may use this to create reasonable objectives and monitor your development over time. You can determine this by completing a fitness assessment or talking to a medical expert.

Participate in regular exercise: One of the best strategies to increase your stamina is to participate in regular exercise. On most days of the week, try to get in at least 30 minutes of moderate-intensity activity, such as walking, cycling, swimming, or dancing.

Including strength training: Exercises that increase muscular mass and cardiovascular performance. At least twice a week, try to add strength training activities.

Concentrate on cardiovascular activity: Increasing your stamina requires cardiovascular exercise. Strive for 150 minutes or more per week of moderately intense aerobic activity, such as brisk walking, cycling, or swimming.

Including interval training: By forcing your body to exert more effort for brief periods of time, interval training can help you increase your stamina. Consider adding brief intervals of intense exercise interspersed with rest or low-intensity activity to your daily regimen.

Boost your nutrition: A healthy diet is crucial for increasing your stamina. Eat a diet that is well-balanced and full of fresh produce, whole grains, lean meats, and healthy fats.

Obtain adequate sleep and recovery time: Increasing your stamina requires getting enough sleep and recovery time. Aim for at least 7-8 hours of sleep every night, and give your body time to recuperate after working out.

Maintaining hydration is important because as we age, our bodies become less adept at maintaining fluid balance, which can result in dehydration. In order to maintain maximum physical function and increase stamina, it's crucial to stay hydrated. Try to consume at least 8 glasses of water each day, and more if you are exercising.

Including flexibility training: As we just discussed, as you become older, flexibility declines, which can restrict your range of motion and reduce your stamina. Yoga or Pilates-style flexibility exercises can assist increase joint mobility and lower the chance of injury.

Track your development: Tracking your development is crucial for maintaining motivation and attaining your fitness objectives. Maintain a record of your workout regimen, including the kind, length, and level of difficulty, and see how your stamina evolves over time.

As you become older, your body might need a different kind of exercise or a different amount of intensity to maintain its peak fitness. It's crucial to be adaptable and vary your schedule as necessary to take into account physical changes.

Get expert advice: It's crucial to seek advice from a healthcare provider or qualified personal trainer if you're new to exercising or if you have any underlying medical concerns. They can assist you in creating a safe and efficient fitness plan that is customized to your unique requirements and capabilities.

As a result, maintaining your stamina as you age calls for a multifaceted strategy that includes consistent physical activity, strength training, cardiovascular exercise, flexibility training, good nutrition, hydration, rest and recovery, monitoring your progress, and seeking professional advice as necessary. You may increase your endurance, lower your chance of developing chronic illnesses, and enhance your general quality of life by implementing these techniques into your daily practice.

CHAPTER TWO

It's crucial to assess your level of fitness before starting to increase your stamina. You will be given the tools in this chapter to evaluate your current stamina level and choose the best place to start your stamina improvement adventure.

Fitness Evaluations

Fitness evaluations are a terrific approach to find out your current level of endurance. Personal trainers, doctors, or other healthcare professionals can carry out these evaluations. Below are a few typical fitness tests that are used to gauge stamina:

Cardiovascular endurance: This examination evaluates the effectiveness with which your heart and lungs can supply oxygen to your working muscles. The step test, stationary bike test, and treadmill test are examples of common assessments.

Muscular endurance: This test determines how many repetitions of an activity you can carry out before becoming fatigued, or how long you can maintain a muscle contraction. Push-ups, sit-ups, and the plank test are typical assessments.

Flexibility: This test evaluates the range of motion in your body's joints. The sit-and-reach test and the shoulder flexibility test are typical assessments.

Body composition: This test calculates your body's proportion of lean muscle, bone, and fat. Skinfold measures, bioelectrical impedance, and dual-energy x-ray absorptiometry (DEXA) scans are examples of typical examinations.

Self-Assessments

There are a number of self-assessments you may carry out to gauge your current level of stamina if you do not have access to a healthcare provider or fitness trainer. These are a few instances:

Test your walking speed by covering a certain distance—say, a mile or a block—while keeping track of your time. Keep track of the duration and the aftereffects.

Pace your ascent of a flight of steps, such as those in your home or a local park, to do the stair test. Keep track of how many flights you can ascend and your post-climb mood.

Test your balance by standing on one foot as long as you can without tipping over. Repeat with the opposite foot, noting how long you can maintain the posture.

Test your ability to breathe deeply by focusing on how long you can hold each deep breath before becoming out of breath or exhausted.

Analyzing the Findings

It's critical to evaluate the findings of your fitness assessment in light of your overall health and fitness objectives. When starting any new fitness program, it is crucial to discuss your findings with your healthcare practitioner if you have any underlying medical concerns, such as high blood pressure or arthritis.

Don't be disheartened if your findings show that your current level of stamina is less than you would like it to be. It is never too late to begin making improvements to your health. You may increase your endurance and reach your ideal level of physical fitness by engaging in regular physical activity, strength training, cardiovascular exercise, flexibility training, good nutrition, hydration, rest and recuperation, and tracking your progress.

Keep in mind that your age and gender might have an impact on your performance when interpreting the results of your fitness testing. For instance, it is typical for women to do worse on tests of physical endurance than males because of variations in muscle mass and hormone levels. Due to age-related changes in the cardiovascular system, older people may also do worse on tests of cardiovascular endurance.

It's crucial to concentrate on your own development throughout time rather than comparing your outcomes to those of others. Your objective should be to increase your level of fitness and achieve your own health objectives.

It's also critical to remember that fitness evaluations are not always accurate indicators of overall health and fitness. They give a momentary glimpse of your physical capabilities, but they do not always represent your overall health. Overall health and well-being are influenced by a number of other variables, including mental health, diet, and lifestyle choices.

Lastly, it's crucial to take into account your general quality of life while assessing your current degree of endurance. How do you feel all day long? Do you have the energy necessary to go through your everyday duties without becoming tired? Can you engage in the things you like without feeling constrained by your physical capabilities? These elements are crucial for determining how fit and healthy you are overall.

Assessing your current degree of endurance is a crucial first step in creating a customized fitness program. Always consider your age, gender, and general health objectives when interpreting your results, and keep your attention on your personal development over time. Fitness tests provide you a quick glimpse of your physical capabilities, but many different things affect your overall health and happiness. You may increase your endurance and reach your ideal level of physical fitness by adopting a comprehensive approach to health and fitness.

CHAPTER THREE

Exercise is essential for preserving our health and wellbeing, especially as we become older. Cardiovascular health, muscular strength and endurance, flexibility, balance, and general quality of life can all be enhanced by regular physical activity. We'll offer some fundamental fitness tips for women over 70 in this chapter to support them in continuing to lead active, healthy lives.

It is crucial to speak with your doctor before beginning any new workout regimen to be sure that doing so will not put you at risk. The following exercises can be included into your everyday regimen as soon as your doctor has given you the all-clear.

Activity that raises your heart rate and breathing rate is referred to as cardiovascular exercise, sometimes referred to as aerobic exercise. It is critical for preserving cardiovascular health and can enhance overall stamina. For women over 70, brisk walking, swimming, cycling, dancing, and low-impact aerobics are all advised cardiovascular workouts.

Strength Training: Maintaining muscular strength and endurance is crucial for enhancing total functional capacity and lowering the risk of falls. Squats, lunges, and pushups, as well as resistance band exercises, mild weightlifting, and bodyweight workouts are all recommended for women over the age of 70.

Flexibility Training: Maintaining healthy joint mobility and lowering the risk of injury need flexibility training. Stretching activities including sitting forward folds, seated spinal twists, and hip flexor stretches are advised for women over 70 who want to increase their flexibility.

Balancing training: Maintaining general functional capacity and lowering the risk of falls need balance training. For women over 70, heel-to-toe walking, chair yoga, and standing on one foot are all advised balancing exercises.

Core Training: Maintaining excellent posture, lowering the risk of back discomfort, and enhancing general functional ability all depend on core training. Pelvic tilts, planks, and sitting twists are suggested core workouts for women over 70.

It's crucial to begin a fitness routine initially and progressively increase the intensity and length over time. It's crucial to pay attention to your body's signals and stop exercising if you feel any pain or discomfort.

It is essential to remember that each person's talents and goals should be taken into account while designing an exercise regimen. If a woman over the age of 70 has never exercised regularly, she may need to begin with lower-intensity activities and progressively raise the intensity over time. While designing an exercise regimen, it's crucial to consider any physical restrictions or existing medical concerns.

Women over 70 should emphasis remaining active throughout the day in addition to the specialized activities mentioned above. This might involve undertaking tasks like gardening, dog walking, or choosing the stairs over the elevator. Regular physical activity helps preserve general physical function and lower the chance of developing chronic illnesses.

When participating in physical exercise, it's equally crucial to give priority to relaxation and rehabilitation. For appropriate recuperation, women over 70 may need to take additional days off between workouts. A healthy diet and adequate sleep are other factors that can enhance fitness recovery and general well-being.

It's critical to make exercise fun and enduring. Making fitness a habit and adding fun activities into a regular schedule can promote long-term success. Finding an exercise partner or enrolling in a group fitness class may also assist with accountability and support.

The fundamental workout suggestions for women over 70 should consist of cardio, strength, flexibility, balance, and core exercises. Together with regular activity, appropriate relaxation, and recovery, these exercises should be tailored to each person's skills and goals. Ensuring long-term success as well as general health and well-being may be accomplished by making exercise fun and enduring.

CHAPTER THREE

While physical activity is necessary for building stamina, a healthy diet is equally critical for preserving energy levels and maintaining general physical health. In this chapter, we will examine how nutrition affects the development of stamina and offer suggestions for a wholesome, well-balanced diet that will help this process.

Macronutrients: Macronutrients give the body energy and are necessary for sustaining stamina. They include carbs, protein, and fat. The body uses carbohydrates as its main energy source, which should account for 45–65% of daily caloric intake. In contrast to simple carbs, which can lead to energy crashes, complex carbohydrates, such as those found in whole grains, fruits, and vegetables, offer continuous energy. Protein should account for 10 to 35% of daily caloric intake since it is crucial for maintaining and rebuilding muscular tissue. Protein may be found in lean meats, fish, beans, and nuts. Furthermore essential for energy, fat should account for 20–35% of daily caloric intake. Olive oil, avocados, nuts, seeds, and seeds are among the sources of good fats.

Micronutrients: Vitamins, minerals, and other micronutrients are crucial for preserving general health and energy levels. Animal items including meat, eggs, and dairy products include vitamin B12, which is necessary for the creation of energy. Red meat, beans, and dark leafy greens are just a few examples of foods that are rich in iron, which is necessary for the body's oxygen transport system. Magnesium, which is included in foods like nuts, seeds, and leafy greens, is crucial for sustaining energy levels.

Hydration: Being well hydrated is essential for preserving energy and avoiding weariness. Women over 70 should try to consume at least 8 glasses of water each day, and more if they are exercising. Fruits and vegetables, soups with broth, and herbal teas are other sources of hydration.

Timing of meals: Eating at the right times can assist maintain energy levels and prevent weariness. Eating modest, frequent meals throughout the day can help manage blood sugar levels and prevent energy dumps. Before exercising, eating a balanced meal with carbs, protein, and fat can also aid to offer long-lasting energy.

Supplements: Although eating a healthy, balanced diet is the best way to get all the nutrients you need, taking supplements can still help you stay energetic. Iron, magnesium, and vitamin B12 supplements can boost the creation of energy and lessen exhaustion.

It is significant to remember that dietary requirements might change depending on a person's age, weight, height, amount of physical activity, and medical issues. Individual dietary needs can be satisfied by seeking advice from a medical expert or qualified dietitian.

To getting the right nutrition, it's critical to avoid bad behaviors that might harm your health in general and your energy levels in particular. Limiting or abstaining from alcohol, cigarettes, processed meals, and high-sugar foods are all part of this.

Consuming a nutritious, balanced diet has many positive health effects in addition to promoting the development of stamina. The chance of developing chronic conditions including heart disease, diabetes, and certain malignancies is decreased, and the quality of life and mental health are also improved.

It can be difficult to incorporate good eating habits into daily life, but there are ways that can assist. This involves preparing meals at home, meal planning, and looking for wholesome substitutes for bad foods. Healthy eating can also be made easier to maintain by asking for assistance from friends, family, or a healthcare professional.

Sustaining general health and wellbeing for women over 70, as well as promoting the development of stamina, requires correct diet. Avoiding bad behaviors and eating a good, balanced diet that includes water, macronutrients, and micronutrients will assist boost energy levels and prevent weariness. Women over 70 can increase their stamina and experience a greater quality of life by implementing healthy eating habits into their everyday lives.

CHAPTER FOUR

The capacity of the heart, lungs, and circulatory system to provide oxygen and nutrients to the muscles while engaging in physical exercise is known as cardiovascular endurance. This is crucial for general stamina and physical fitness since it enables people to exercise for extended periods of time without getting tired. We will examine exercises that improve cardiovascular endurance in this chapter and offer suggestions for adopting these exercises into daily living.

Aerobic Exercise : Activity that raises heart rate and breathing rate is referred to as aerobic exercise and includes activities like walking, jogging, cycling, and swimming. By enhancing the functionality of the heart, lungs, and circulatory system, these exercises can assist build cardiovascular endurance. Adults should engage in at least 150 minutes of moderate-intensity aerobic activity or 75 minutes of vigorous-intensity aerobic activity per week, according to the American Heart Association.

High-Intensity Interval Training (HIIT): This is a kind of exercise that alternates brief bursts of high intensity with rest or lower level activity. It has been demonstrated that this form of exercise increases the heart's and circulatory system's effectiveness, hence enhancing cardiovascular endurance. Running, cycling, and bodyweight movements are all examples of HIIT exercises.

Circuit Training: In circuit training, a number of exercises are performed one after the other with little rest in between. By raising heart rate and giving the entire body a workout, this form of exercise can enhance cardiovascular endurance. Exercises that require little to no equipment, such as resistance bands or weights, are also suitable for circuit training.

Dancing: Increasing cardiovascular endurance via dancing is enjoyable and beneficial. Dancing may be done in a number of forms, such as ballroom, salsa, or Zumba, and incorporates movements that speed up the heart rate and breathing rate.

Sports: Playing sports like tennis, basketball, or soccer can increase cardiovascular endurance by boosting heart rate and giving the entire body a workout. Sports' social component can also enhance the enjoyment and motivation of exercise.

It's crucial to begin at a comfortable level while engaging in activities that develop cardiovascular endurance and to progressively increase intensity and duration over time. This can lessen the risk of injury and raise general fitness levels. When beginning a new workout regimen, it's also crucial to speak with a healthcare provider, especially if there are any underlying medical concerns.

Increasing cardiovascular endurance through exercise is a crucial part of total vigor and physical health for women over 70. Cardiovascular endurance may be improved by aerobic exercise, HIIT, circuit training, dance, and sports, all of which can be introduced into everyday life in different ways. Women over 70 can increase their cardiovascular endurance and benefit from the many health advantages of regular physical exercise by gradually increasing intensity and duration, working with a healthcare practitioner, and exercising regularly.

CHAPTER FOUR

Working against resistance is a sort of exercise that helps maintain and increase muscular growth and strength. By boosting muscular performance and enhancing general fitness, this kind of exercise can also increase stamina. In this chapter, we'll look at the advantages of strength training for building stamina and offer suggestions on how to integrate it into your regular routine.

Women over 70 can enhance their stamina through strength training to a great extent. We naturally start to lose muscular mass and strength as we get older, which might affect our stamina and quality of life. By maintaining and gaining muscle mass and strength, raising bone density, and enhancing metabolic process, strength training can help slow down this natural decrease.

Improved cardiovascular endurance is one of the main advantages of strength training for the development of stamina. Strength training can help the body utilise oxygen more effectively by improving the efficiency of the muscles and circulatory system, enabling longer and more sustained physical activity. Older folks, who may be more susceptible to cardiovascular disease and other chronic diseases, may find this to be of particular importance.

Strength training can help promote general physical fitness and physical endurance in daily activities. This can lead to better flexibility, balance, and coordination as well as more power and stamina. Women over 70 can keep their independence and enhance their quality of life by increasing their total physical fitness.

Exercises for Strengthening,

Bodyweight exercises, resistance band exercises, and weightlifting are just a few of the several strength training activities that may be done to increase endurance.

Exercises with resistance bands, which may be performed at the gym or at home, employ elastic bands to produce resistance. Leg extensions, shoulder presses, and bicep curls are a few examples of resistance band workouts. Depending on each person's degree of fitness, the resistance for these exercises can be changed.

Weightlifting is working against resistance while utilizing free weights or weight machines. With the appropriate equipment, this kind of strength training may be performed at home or at a gym. Bench presses, deadlifts, and squats are a few types of weightlifting exercises. Weightlifting exercises should be performed with good form and technique to minimize injury risk and enhance workout efficacy.

Duration and Recurrence

Depending on the demands and objectives of each person, the frequency and length of strength training sessions might change. Beginners are advised to begin with one or two sessions per week that last 20 to 30 minutes each. Frequency and length can be increased as fitness levels rise.

For older folks in particular, it's crucial to provide enough time for rest and recuperation in between strength training sessions. In addition to giving the muscles time to recuperate and expand, this can assist avoid injury.

Proper technique and form

To avoid injuries and maximize the benefits of strength training exercises, it is crucial to do them with the correct form and technique. This might involve maintaining a straight back, using the entire range of motion, and contracting the core muscles.

While beginning strength training, it's crucial to use lesser weights or less resistance and to concentrate on utilizing appropriate form and technique before introducing more resistance or difficulty.

Development and Variety

It's critical to gradually raise the resistance or intensity of the workouts and include variation in the program to keep stamina gains going and prevent plateaus. To achieve this, you can lift heavier weights, perform more repetitions, or try out new exercises.

Variety in a strength training regimen may also aid in avoiding boredom and maintaining desire. This might entail experimenting with various workouts, changing the quantity of sets and repetitions, or utilizing various pieces of kit.

Ladies over 70 can increase their stamina via strength exercise. Strength training can boost overall physical fitness and stamina by increasing muscle mass and strength, bone density, and metabolic function. Resistance training with a band

CHAPTER FIVE

Popular exercise regimens like yoga and pilates can enhance older women's health in a variety of ways. Both exercises are easy on the body since they emphasize regulated movements, in-depth breathing, and awareness. The advantages of yoga and Pilates for women over 70 are examined in this chapter, along with some of the greatest postures and workouts for enhancing flexibility, balance, and stamina.

Yoga Benefits for Women Over 70

Improved flexibility, balance, strength, and mental wellness are just a few of the numerous health advantages of yoga, an age-old practice. Yoga can be particularly helpful for preserving mobility and lowering the risk of falls for women over the age of 70.

Balance-enhancing yoga postures like tree pose and warrior III can enhance stability and reduce the risk of falling. Posture variations that emphasize flexibility, such the sitting forward fold and the downward dog, help increase range of motion and avoid stiffness. In addition, postures that emphasize strength, like plank and boat pose, can aid in muscle growth and enhance general physical fitness.

Moreover, yoga has been demonstrated to enhance mental health by lowering stress, anxiety, and sadness. Yoga may be a helpful technique for enhancing mental wellbeing and raising general quality of life for women over 70 who may be dealing with the difficulties of aging.

Pilates Benefits for Women Over 70

Pilates is a low-impact form of exercise that emphasizes developing stamina, flexibility, and strength. It is a great kind of exercise for women over 70 since it stresses regulated movements, deep breathing, and a strong core.

Pilates can aid with posture, stability, and balance, which can lower the chance of falling and increase mobility in general. Also, it can aid in increasing strength and stamina, making daily tasks easier and less exhausting such as carrying groceries or climbing stairs.

Women over 70 who may be struggling with chronic diseases like osteoporosis or arthritis may find Pilates to be extremely helpful. Pilates can help decrease pain and inflammation while enhancing general physical fitness by emphasizing controlled movements and avoiding high-impact workouts.

Posture and exercise suggestions for yoga and pilates for women over 70

It's crucial for women over 70 to select yoga and Pilates postures and exercises that are suitable for their level of physical condition and capabilities. These are some positions and exercises that are advised:

Mountain position in yoga

A tree posture

Soldier III

Backward dog

sitting forward-folding the bridge stance

Exercises for Pilates: Pelvic tilt

Leg rotations

Roll-ups

lateral leg raises

Sword kicks

spinal extension

While starting yoga or Pilates, it's crucial to work with a trained teacher or physical therapist, especially if you have any ongoing medical issues or physical restrictions.

Advice for Beginning Yoga and Pilates

These are a few pointers to get you started if you want to attempt yoga or Pilates:

begin slowly: Work your way up to more advanced postures and exercises starting with beginner-level courses or exercises.

Emphasis on form: To avoid injury and maximize the benefits of the exercise, proper form and technique are crucial.

Observe your body: Stop doing the posture or exercise if it makes you feel pain or discomfort and get advice from a licensed teacher or physical therapist.

Be stable and reliable: When it comes to yoga and Pilates, consistency is crucial. For best results, try to practice at least once or twice every week.

Enjoy yourself: Pilates and yoga should be pleasurable! Find what works best for you by experimenting with various stances and workouts.

In conclusion, there are several health advantages of yoga and pilates.

CHAPTER SIX

Women who are older may discover that they still like certain pastimes or occupations that call for a certain amount of power and endurance. Having a strong physique may make activities like gardening, playing with the grandkids, or traveling more fun and less strenuous. This chapter will discuss a few unique strengthening exercises that can assist women over 70 perform better in certain tasks.

Gardening

Women over the age of 70 like gardening, but it may be physically taxing. It takes some power and endurance to do things like digging, planting, and weeding. There are a number of strengthening exercises that may be performed to enhance gardening performance:

Squats: Squats may increase leg strength, which is beneficial for activities like bending and lifting.

Lunges: Lunges can enhance stability and balance, which is beneficial for negotiating uneven terrain.

Deadlifts: Deadlifts may strengthen the lower back and the core, which is useful for jobs like lifting mulch or soil bags.

interacting with grandkids

Although though playing with grandkids may be enjoyable and gratifying, it can also be physically taxing. It may be necessary to have a particular amount of strength and stamina to run, leap, and lift. There are numerous strengthening exercises that may be done to enhance performance when playing with grandchildren:

Squats: Squats can improve leg strength, which is beneficial for activities like lifting and carrying young children.

Push-ups: These exercises may strengthen your upper body, which is beneficial for jobs like scooping up your grandchildren.

Planks: When playing with the grandkids, keeping balance and stability may be made easier by strengthening the core.

Traveling

Although while it may be a thrilling adventure, traveling can be physically taxing. A certain amount of strength and endurance may be needed for carrying heavy loads, covering long distances on foot, and negotiating challenging terrain. There are a number of strengthening exercises that may be done to enhance performance when traveling:

Squats: Squats can improve leg strength, which is beneficial for carrying heavy loads and strenuous walking.

Lunges: Lunges can enhance stability and balance, which is beneficial for negotiating uneven terrain.

Presses on the shoulders: Presses on the shoulders can develop upper body strength, which is beneficial for carrying luggage.

Suggestions for Building Strength for Specific Activities

It's crucial to keep in mind a few guidelines to maintain your health and safety when participating in certain activities:

begin slowly: Start with a beginner's fitness regimen and progress to increasingly difficult activities over time.

Emphasis on form: To avoid injury and maximize the benefits of the exercise, proper form and technique are crucial.

Pay attention to your body: If an activity makes you uncomfortable or in pain, stop and get advice from a certified trainer or physical therapist.

Be dependable: When it comes to strengthening for certain activities, consistency is essential. For best results, try to practice at least once or twice every week.

Having fun: Building up your strength for a certain activity should be pleasurable! Choose workouts that are enjoyable and stimulating, and concentrate on the things you want to do.

Finally, strengthening exercises may be specifically designed for particular activities to enable women over 70 both perform better and take part in their preferred hobbies and interests. You may increase your strength and endurance and make doing daily activities simpler and more pleasant by concentrating on the workouts that are most pertinent to your interests.

CONCLUSION

For any woman over the age of 70 who wants to increase her stamina, energy, and general health, "70-Year-Old Women's Stamina Development" is a helpful resource. The book covers a wide range of subjects, including fundamental workout suggestions, nutrition, strength training, aerobic activity, and specific strengthening exercises for certain occupations. It offers helpful advice and simple directions. Women over 70 may take charge of their health, increase their vitality, and enjoy a greater quality of life by heeding the suggestions in this book.